Sherlock Has Th

Written By: Adrienne [Reade]

Illustrated By: Brandy Roy & Mandy Morreale

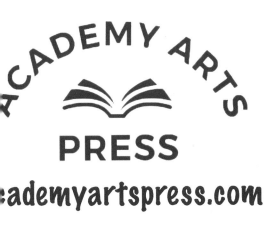

academyartspress.com

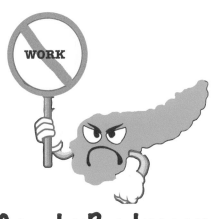

CrankyPanky.com

Hi! My name is London and
this is my dog Sherlock.
I have Type 1 Diabetes and Sherlock is my
highly trained Diabetic Alert Dog.
He's also my best friend and
he goes everywhere I go.

1

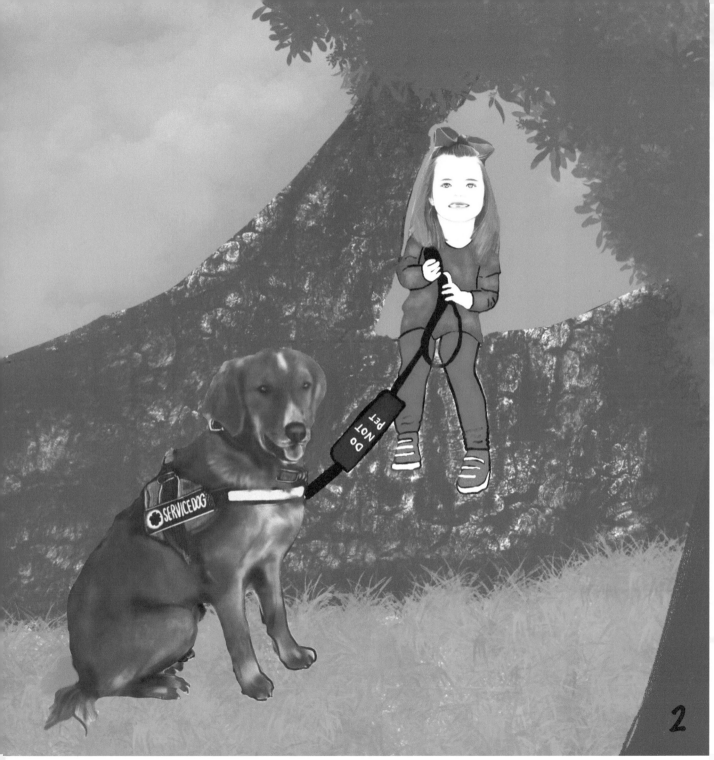

2

When I was only 16-months old,
I was diagnosed with T1D.
It was a huge shock and
my parents were very worried.
I was so young that I wasn't able to tell
them how I was feeling.
My blood sugar could drop dangerously low
or spike very high with no warning.

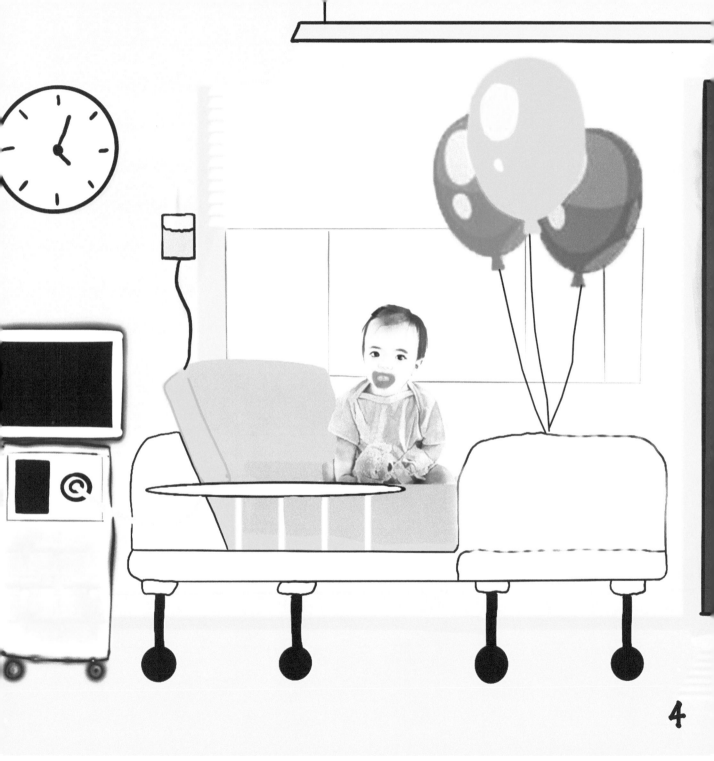

Luckily for us, a very special puppy had
just been born. Little did we know
he was going to be my
lifesaving dog one day!

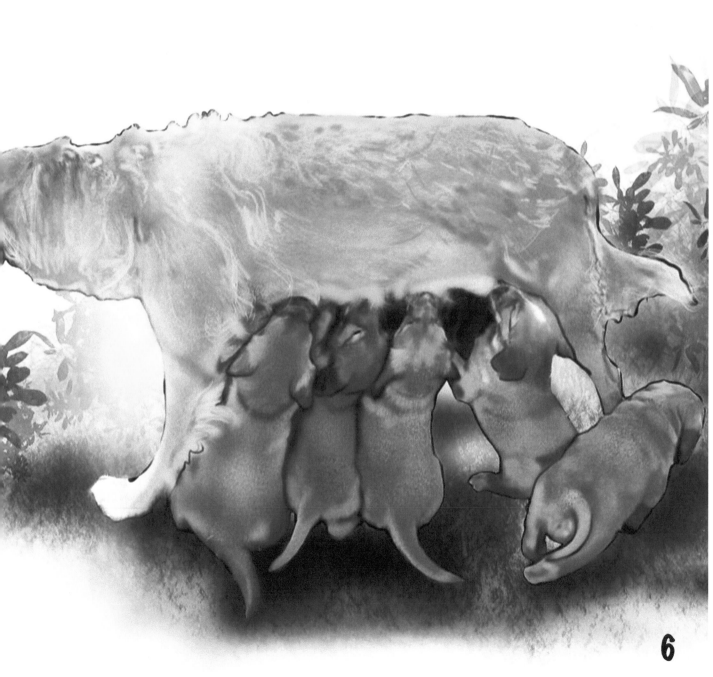

My parents researched all they could about T1D and found out that dogs can smell changes in blood sugar with amazing accuracy. We found an organization in our area who trained Diabetic Alert dogs and started the process of getting one.

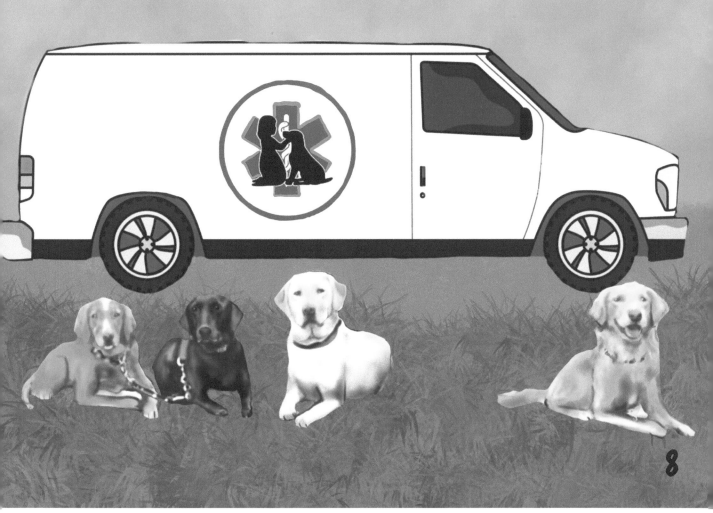

Meanwhile, those puppies were growing
up and one had a white blaze on his nose,
and chest, and was born
with the cutest short tail.
He was chosen to go California to meet a
special little girl.

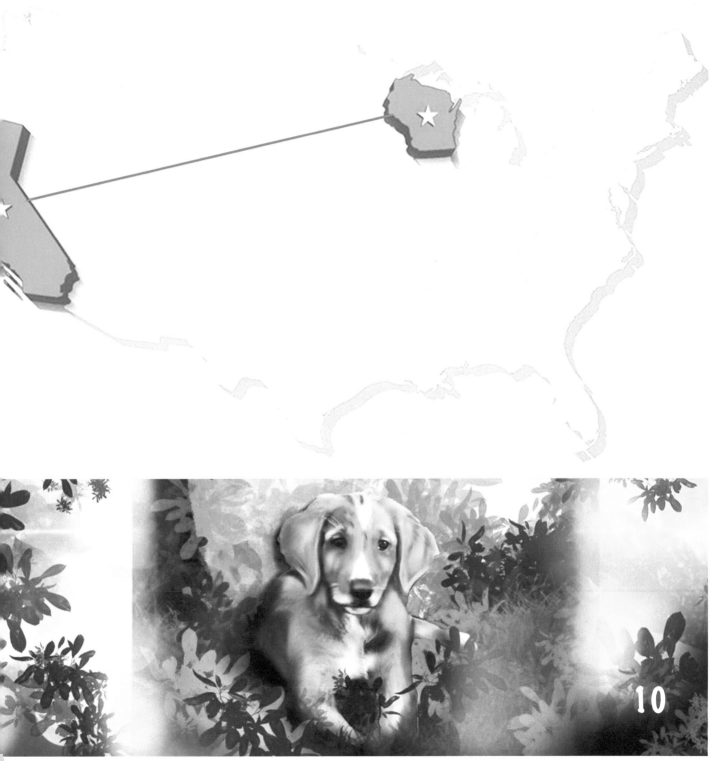

We tried working with a few dogs until our trainer found the perfect fit for my family and me.
You can't really get any more perfect, because Sherlock was named before he was placed with me.

Although it's quite fitting isn't it?!
Sherlock is a blood sugar detective!

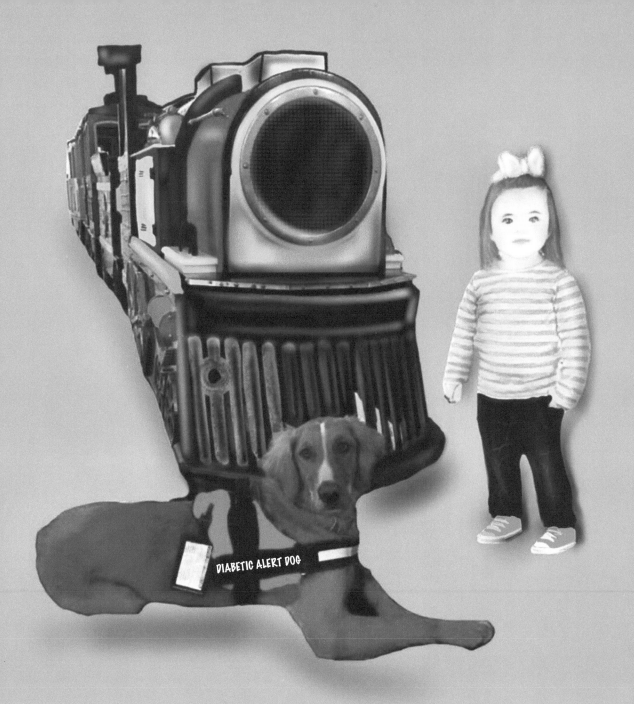

DIABETIC ALERT DOG

12

It took nearly two years of waiting to get
placed with our forever dog.
Diabetic Alert Dogs are very specialized
and their training is expensive.

We did a T-Shirt fundraiser to raise money
and spread awareness about
T1D and Sherlock.

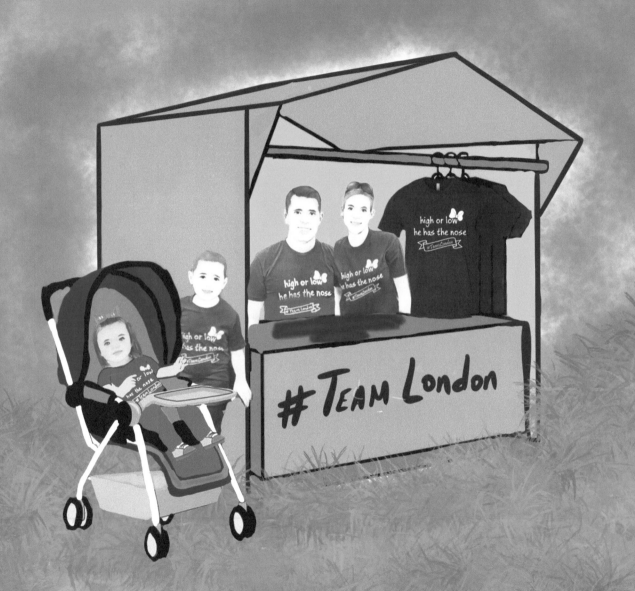

When we got Sherlock home the real work began. He was trained to be a Diabetic Alert dog, but we needed to learn how to be good handlers.
That included learning how a service dog should behave in public, and how to react to Sherlock and his alerts.
It was hard at first...lots of extra finger sticks and reinforcing what we wanted Sherlock to do.

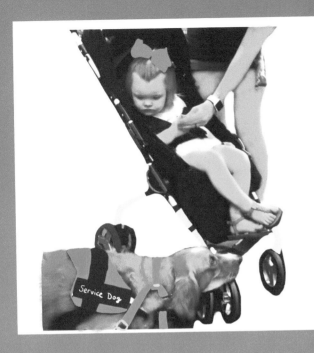

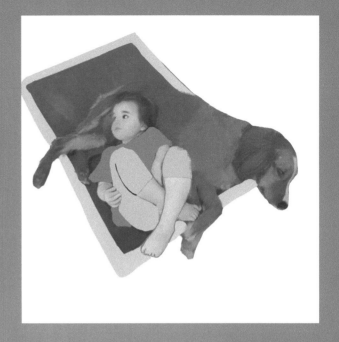

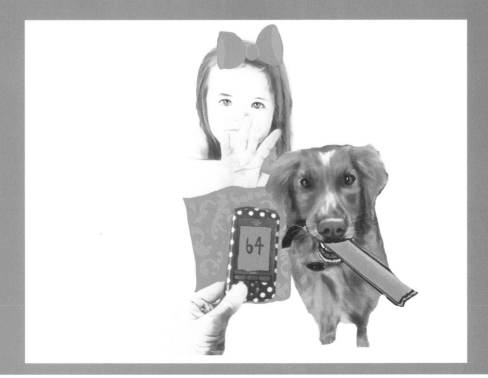

16

Sherlock can smell when my blood sugar goes too low or too high. He retrieves a dog training bringsel and brings it to my Mom or Dad. When he alerts us, we test my blood sugar by pricking my finger to see if he is right.
I wear a blood glucose monitor as well but Sherlock is usually faster than the monitor...
Always trust the nose!

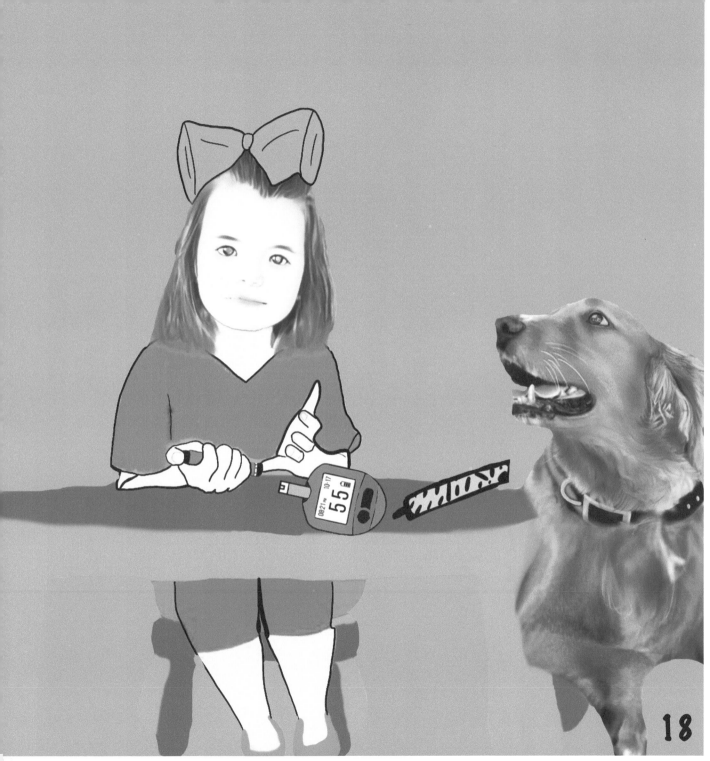

18

When Sherlock alerts and tells us that my blood
sugar is out of range he gets a "puppy party!"
That's a treat, a toy, or a chance to
play ball or tug outside.

I also scratch or pet him and tell him what a good boy
he is! He works hard, but plays hard too!
He gets to nap in his crate for a few hours
each day because T1D is tiring!

My mom wonders why she doesn't
get to take a nap too?

19

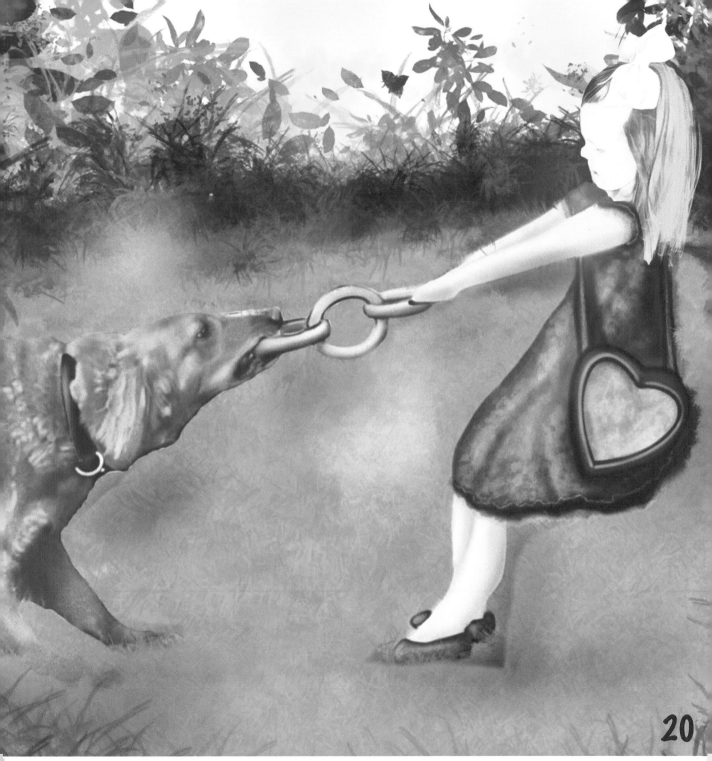

20

Some people might think that my Mom and Dad
sleep better having Sherlock around.
While he does keep me safe at night he also
wakes up my parents to tell them
about a low or high...
Even at 2 AM!
It's all worth it though, because he has saved
my life countless times.

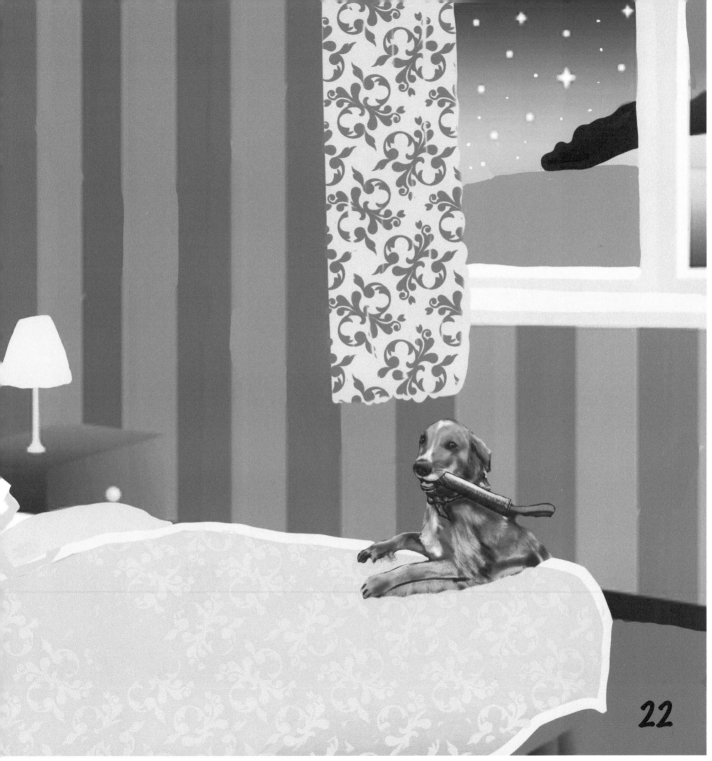

It may look like fun to take your dog everywhere, but it's a lot of extra work and responsibility! People ask if they can pet Sherlock and I have to explain to them that he is working.

Sherlock always behaves well in public and that's a very important part of being a service dog. When we go out we make sure we bring Sherlock's bringsel, treats, water, and food for longer trips, and his shoes to protect his feet when it's hot out.

Have you ever seen a dog wearing shoes?
Lots of comments when people see that !

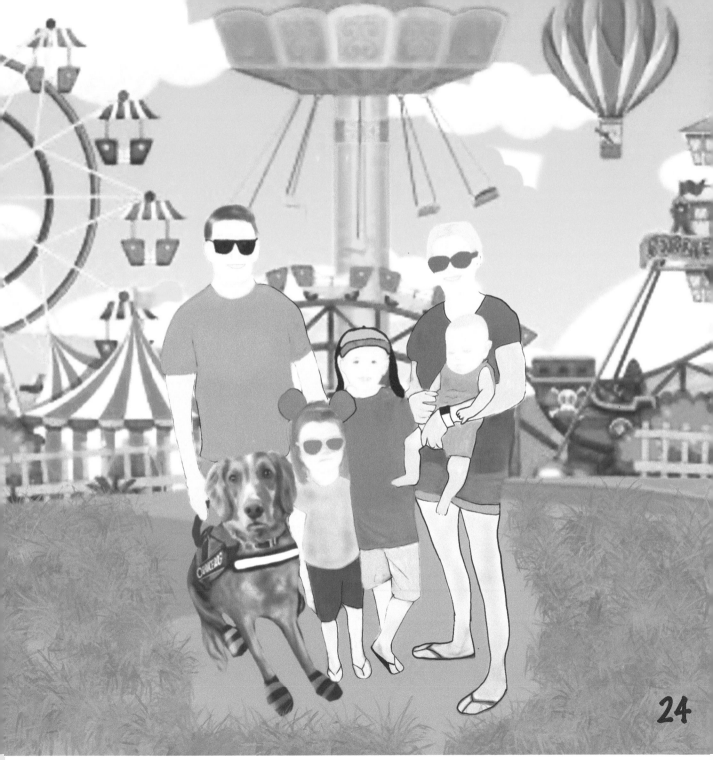

24

Sherlock is highly trained, but he can miss an
alert here and there....
Sometimes he just wants to play.
Don't we all?!

However, most of the time his alerts
are spot on and he loves to work!

He is great at cuddling or giving me a kiss if
I'm not feeling great, like when my blood sugar
is out of range.

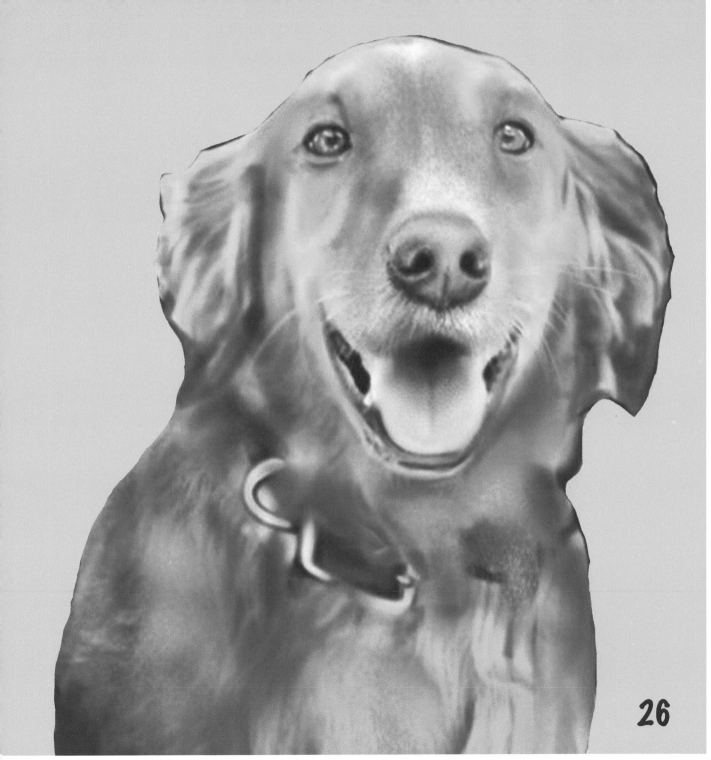

26

Sherlock is so much more than just a dog to me.
I am so lucky to have him.
He truly is my best friend, and a real lifesaver!

I love you, Sherlock!

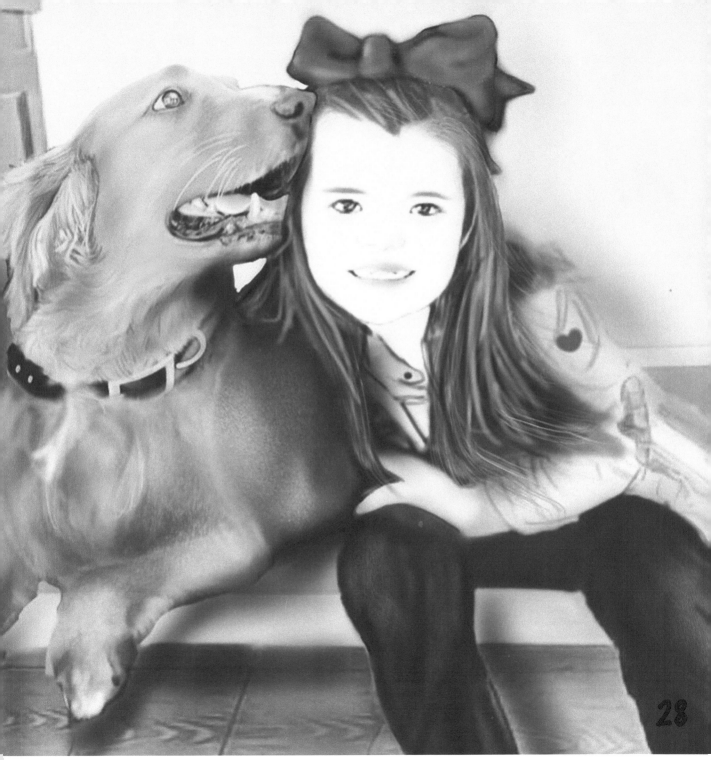

To follow our journey, or to learn more about London and Sherlock please follow us on Facebook and Instagram - TeamLondonT1D

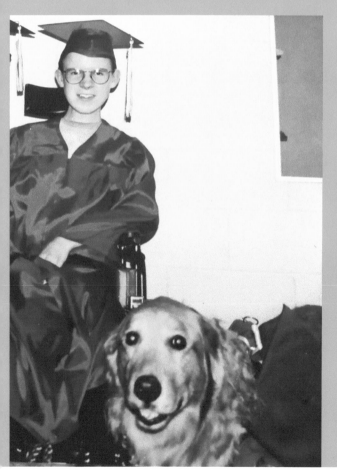

In loving memory of my Brother John Lanspery. He would have been very proud of this book and our educating others about service dogs.
John had a Canine Companion service do Newman, who helped him with his Duchenne Muscular Dystrophy diagnosis We dedicate this book to you, John!

CPSIA information can be obtained
at www.ICGtesting.com
Printed in the USA
LVHW071935170521
687671LV00003B/5

9781087965994